Salty
For Beginners

The Beginners Step By Step Guide To Creating And Keeping A Stunning Saltwater Aquarium Using The Expert Skills

Dr. Danny Bryan

Table of Contents

CHAPTER ONE 3

   Saltwater Aquariums 3

CHAPTER TWO 30

   Do fish develop to the tank size of theirs?...30

   Is saltwater more complex?........................32

   Just how much experience do I need?.........36

CHAPTER THREE 41

   The Innovative Marine Nuvo 41

CHAPTER ONE

Saltwater Aquariums

A contemporary saltwater aquarist is not dependent on tailor container companies to develop professional quality tanks, ideal for a saltwater merrell. You are able to actually pick from a huge selection of various aquariums of all the sizes and shapes, and also have a single delivered to the doorstep of yours inside just a couple times. From all-in-one tanks as well as nano cubes to significantly bigger show tanks finish with an overflow package and sump.

Not merely has got the choice developed right away within the last 10 20 yrs, though we've additionally observed characteristics such as low iron cup, aluminum framed container stands, along with experienced filtration actually raise the industrial aquariums attainable to household aquarists.

The truth is, in case you wish to attain long-lasting

accomplishment, you have to select the aquarium which is appropriate for you as well as the lifestyle of yours. This very helpful Buyer 's Guide can help go with you with the toilet tank which very best fits the aquarium goals of yours. You are able to additionally shop by tank size or maybe product when exploring the entire catalog of ours of aquariums.

- For The Dorm, Apartment, Or perhaps Otherwise Space

Starved: Innovative Marine Nuvo Fusion ten Pro and Advanced Acrylics Pico and Nano Cube

• For The Creative Workspace: Innovative Marine Concept Drop Off or perhaps Concept Encore

• For The Countertop: Innovative Marine Nuvo Fusion Peninsula or perhaps Fiji Cube twenty Gallon AIO Rimless Peninsula • For The Bookshelf: AquaMaxx twelve

Gallon Long or perhaps Mr. Aqua Bookshelf

• For The Minimalist: AquaMaxx Rimless or perhaps Mr. Aqua Low-Iron

• For The Frag Farmer: Advanced Acrylics Frag Tanks

• For The "Go Big Or perhaps Go Home": Reddish Sea Reefer Deluxe along with Fiji Cube • The brief answer is NO! In days gone by, saltwater aquariums have been considered as being difficult and mysterious to preserve. At the moment which might were correct, but that is not the truth nowadays. The saltwater aquarium pastime consistently produce in recognition because of the improvement of quality tools as well as help solutions, together with a clear understanding of the requirements of marine organisms and the way to offer them. This has led numerous freshwater hobbyists and finish beginners to test the hand of theirs at holding saltwater aquariums.

Creating a saltwater aquarium requires a great deal of work. You will be astonished to discover the number of goods are required to work it. When you've designed what sort of saltwater aquarium you like and bought anything had to assemble it, stick to the guidelines to buy the new marine aquarium of yours operating in a harmless, orderly way.

Create the Aquarium Grab the aquarium completely ready. Place the rise up into level and place it. You'll want to keep clearance for electric equipment and connections. Cleanse the toilet tank with a soft cloth or maybe sponge & work with water that is fresh. Put container backing as well as place the toilet tank on a stand, in case you intend to.

Electrical contacts include: • Sump: If you've elected to

utilize a sump, get it and also the sump related gear in the cabinet/stand. Frequently it's less difficult to place the sump directly into the rise up through the best than it's through the cabinet doors. When you haven't discovered a sump but still, an inexpensive, simple DIY sump may work.

• Top off System: If you're likely to use a DIY automated top off structure, get it done just before you get the sump of yours (it is drastically simpler than patiently waiting until finally the sump is in the cabinet).

• Power strip as well as mild timer

Set up the Sump Equipment
In this phase, you are going to install the sump and its connected plumbing and equipment underneath the aquarium. When you stick to the actions, one at a time, the sump tools fitting goes together really quick. When

you're not employing a sump, bypass the phase.

If perhaps the system of yours works with a sump: 1. Install resources in the wet/dry trickle filter

2. Install the overflow hose pipe from the toilet tank to the sump (pictured, 1)

3. Install the go back pump (pictured, two) and also hose pipe (pictured, 4)

4. Install sump mounted protein-rich skimmer

5. Install aquarium heater

Invest the Aquarium Equipment If the system of yours doesn't use a sump, you are able to start working on setting up the tank related tools. At this stage, you are able to postpone setting up your aquarium lighting program as it'll simply stay in how when you're setting up the sea salts, substrate, and container accents.

Prep the purifier by eliminating the filtration pads,

rinsing them in water that is fresh, consequently placing them also in the purifier before adding it on the rear wall structure of the aquarium. This's a great time to check out the clearance in between the rear of the wall and the tank. You'll be eliminating the whole air filter down the road for cleansing, as ensure that there's an additional inch or perhaps 2 of clearance.

Use the tank mounted air purification system (hang on canister or tank, the tank mounted protein-rich skimmer, and also the powerheads. Dangle the powerheads of yours in the rough place you are going to have them in the conclusion of assembly. The roles will undoubtedly alter once the live rock of yours & accessories are set up on the toilet tank. Set up the aquarium heater.

Run a damp Test of the device Before you place in sea salts, live animals or rock, or maybe substrate, you must operate a system stormy start testing. Choosing the time period to perform this enables you to ensure that all of the contacts as well as tools are in appropriate working order. Majority of damp assessments work with water that is fresh. You don't desire to set up some existing sand or maybe wildlife only at that stage, water that is fresh coming from the damp check is able to destroy each.

1. Check and tighten up all of the hose pipe connections

2. Fill the aquarium (and sump, in case you're utilizing one) with water that is fresh

3. Wipe the outside of the toilet tank and also the complete region dry

4. One at a moment, plug every pump directly into the energy strip

5. Check every plumbing link for leaks

6. If you're likely to be consuming a protein skimmer, there is going to be absolutely no waste created, though you are able to look for bubble generation in addition to test out the pump which are going to be utilized to operate it.

7. Simulate a power outage by switching off of the whole method in the energy strip/timer. In case you're

consuming a sump, ensure it doesn't overflow as the sump pump prevents pumping and also gas tank h2o is siphoned back again into the sump. In case the sump begins to overflow, switch the pump returned on and eliminate several of the drinking water coming from the sump. Reactivate the device and also retest it.

One strategy to avoid siphoning container faucet back in to the sump is drilling a tiny gap in the sump pump go back pipe above the toilet tank water collection in the toilet tank. In the function of any power outage (and each time the go back pump is switched off) the little gap enables the siphon to be reduced.

Insert Sea and Substrate Salts Choosing the proper substrate for the tank of yours prior to setting up it's vital, in case for not one other purpose than it's tough to eliminate after the container is running. Additionally, research in advance and find out probably the very best sea salt for the particular aquarium of yours.

After the method was examined for leaks, shut the device down and eliminate a couple of gallons of h20 out of the toilet tank as well as sump.

Then, put in the sea salts of yours. In case you're consuming a sump, put the sea salts to the sump and switch on the sump return pump. This can flow drinking water with the sea salts and enable them to dissolve faster. When you do not possess a sump, switch on virtually any powerheads in the toilet tank, together with the filter of yours. As the sea salts dissolve, continue adding additional and evaluate the salinity often until finally the preferred amount is covered.

In case you're utilizing living sand, put it within the toilet tank. The bath is going to become cloudy, though it ought to clean up when you've switched on the filtration system of yours. In case you're utilizing non live sand, wash it in water that is fresh to eliminate the smaller sized particles, then put it within the toilet tank.

Situate the Aquascaping and Rock in case you've living rock relieved and all set for usage, or even if perhaps you're not gon na work with living rock at many, you are able to bypass to aquascaping, that is laying out the vegetation, stones, rock, along with other decoration for the toilet tank. When you haven't yet bought living rock and are planning to place a number in the aquarium of yours, this is the time to purchase it and also ready it for usage.

You are able to completely overcome living rock in its own curing established, you are able to cycle the aquarium with living rock, and choose to avoid the rock curing method entirely and place the living rock straight into the aquarium and begin aquascaping.

If perhaps you bypass the curing procedure, it's really suggested you preclean the rubble prior to putting them within the aquarium. Nevertheless, the best case situation is always to preclean the rubble and put them within the aquarium and enable the rubble to completely remedy, and at the very least offer it a couple of days of curing moment just before you aquascape the toilet tank.

Switch on your the, filters, and pumps protein skimmer (in case you're utilizing one). The bath should begin to clean when the screens eliminate the particulate matter in the toilet tank h2o. In many cases, you might envision a facial, practically dust-like coating in addition to the living rubble as well as substrate. These're the nice particles of the substrate which happen to have settled on the bottom part before they might be filtered out. You are able to mix them up with a total deal with or maybe the hand of yours to place them too in to the suspension, that ought to allow the screens to have them out there.

The bath must be apparent by the following day, after which

you could start introducing the critters of yours on the toilet tank.

CHAPTER TWO

Do fish develop to the tank size of theirs?

Several aquarists fall into the hole of "it is only going to develop on the dimensions of my aquarium." This's incorrect - tank measurement doesn't govern what size a fish will have. This particular misconception is the root cause of many undesirable, stunted fish in health that is poor, in addition to a good amount of stressed away fish proprietors. An additional concern is that the majority of Tank Buster species live best more than twenty years, which makes them a long-range dedication for anybody that buys them.

Getting started with a saltwater aquarium: While it's correct the marine aquarium pastime is much more costly compared to freshwater, you are able to begin with a fundamental fish only arrangement & improvement into live corals and invertebrates as the budget of yours and knowledge enable.

Is saltwater more complex?

A bit of. Knowing a couple of additional things about drinking water hormones is crucial to maintaining a saltwater aquarium, though the basics of aquarium to keep are basically exactly the same for new and saltwater.

The secret to accomplishment is going gradually, read

through almost as you are able to and remain inside the means of yours. You will find a lot of methods and techniques for accomplishment, though they do not all job for everybody all of the time. Moreover, blending various pieces and bits of info is able to result in unforeseen outcomes. Find out somebody that has had achievements with saltwater aquariums as well as stick with that individual for guidance up until you get experience that is enough to venture off on ones own.

Purchasing livestock for saltwater aquariums: With regards to purchasing other critters and fish, do the homework of yours! Be sure you comprehend the requirements as well as compatibility of all livestock prior to buying. Quarantine most brand new livestock buys before introducing them to your screen container to stay away from introducing disease organisms.

Gear for saltwater aquariums Begin with the biggest aquarium and also the very best equipment you are able to pay for. Nano tanks do not cost you that much and occupy much less room, but larger aquariums tend to be more steady and much more forgiving of newbie blunders. Do not skimp on the gear of yours! Quality that is good tools is going to perform as promoted as well as hold up as time passes, a thing the animals of yours will definitely value. Be sure you comprehend the skills as well as limitations of all gear just before you create a buy.

Just how much experience do I need?

Despite what several people think, it is not essential to have practical experience with freshwater aquariums before trying saltwater. Marine aquarium to keep involves a bit more patience and a bit more cash than freshwater, but with appropriate research and planning, it is anything that any person is able to do effectively, no matter previous experience.

Remember to work with the newsletter of ours, visit us on Facebook and speak to us for even more info.

For the Dorm, Apartment, Or perhaps Otherwise Space Starved: Innovative Marine Nuvo Fusion ten Pro and

Advanced Acrylics Pico and Nano Cube

A small, square impact along with hundred % integrated filtration have an assortment of advantages for individuals who simply do not have the area or maybe period necessary for a bigger container. These cube shaped tanks are going to fit well upon small countertop or a desk and can simply help support at least one clownfish as well as an anemone or perhaps just several corals and the favorite invertebrates of yours. There's both a glass (Innovative Marine) along with acrylic (Advanced Acrylics) choice thus, in case you're picky, you've alternatives.

The average complete measurement also signifies you will not be spending a large amount of money or time on upkeep and yes it will not need a load of livestock to finish the appearance. Your roommate or friends could easily view the toilet tank when you're from city and also you will not require an additional insurance policy "just in case". Simply being little implies you are able to effortlessly carry things up and move the toilet tank with no multiple trips or extra help also.

CHAPTER THREE

The Innovative Marine Nuvo

Fusion Pro container is basically cup and also has a couple of purification accessories like the required return pump so you are able to spend a lesser amount of time going shopping and much more time experiencing the toilet tank. The Advanced Acrylic Nano and Pico Cubes are produced from clear plastic acrylic plus simply are the bare bones container. You are able to pick from a number of various toilet tank measurements in this particular case; right down to merely a few of gallons. Additionally you get to select the pump along with different filtration add-ons that're sold individually.

As for the last price, you are going to spend a comparable quantity whichever path you go, pick the toilet tank according to the accessible room you've & the preference of yours for whether acrylic or glass.

For any Creative Workspace: Innovative Marine Concept Drop Off or maybe Concept Encore If you recognize originality and love to function as the middle of attention, the tanks are for you. Each provide a really distinctive fabric to make a visually spectacular screen you are going to be satisfied to talk about in the social feed of yours.

drop off tanks imitate the organic merrell drop-off enabling the person to stack rubble in such a manner which produces various zones of equally light and flow in one aquarium. The tanks produce a feeling of depth and permit bad space inside the aquascape of yours which leads to something really different. Its Nuvo Fusion Pro Kit also which means you find the pump and air purification add-ons of the toilet tank. Invest more hours setting up the aquascape of yours as well as a shorter time stressing about other equipment and filtration.

The idea Encore is really the very first of the kind of its, at minimum in the method of commercially available tanks. Every one of the side-by-side screen tanks is independently filtered signifying the tanks won't discuss the identical h2o. You can possibly continue a freshwater placed tank right alongside a saltwater merrell toilet tank for a remarkably contrasting screen.

For the Countertop: Innovative Marine Nuvo Fusion Peninsula or maybe Fiji Cube twenty Gallon AIO Rimless Peninsula These peninsula style tanks are completely formed for positioning on the kitchen counter of yours and supply 3 looking at panes for any 180° perspective into the toilet tank. Built-in purification would mean you will not need to contemplate what sort of purification can be used and will maintain the thoroughly clean appearance, with no anything dangling from the toilet tank.

A 20 gallon container this way will be the ideal size for first time toilet tank proprietors or perhaps people who simply want to maintain cost and maintenance under control. The very long design maximizes the swim room and looking at area for the aquatic pets of yours and also enables you to create a horizontal scape which comments encrusting corals or perhaps freshwater plant life.

Made in United States
North Haven, CT
21 December 2022